SimpleGuy Diet 2

a new and improved look at

A STUBBORN MAN'S MOST *UNEXPECTED* SUCCESS STORY

WRITTEN BY SKIP LEI

ILLUSTRATED BY NITYA WAKHLU

Copyright © 2010, 2013 Skip Lei.

All rights reserved. No part of this book may be reproduced, stored, or transmitted by any means—whether auditory, graphic, mechanical, or electronic—without written permission of both publisher and author, except in the case of brief excerpts used in critical articles and reviews. Unauthorized reproduction of any part of this work is illegal and is punishable by law.

ISBN: 978-1-4834-0203-1 (sc)
ISBN: 978-1-4834-0202-4 (e)

www.simpleguydiet.com

Because of the dynamic nature of the Internet, any web addresses or links contained in this book may have changed since publication and may no longer be valid. The views expressed in this work are solely those of the author and do not necessarily reflect the views of the publisher, and the publisher hereby disclaims any responsibility for them.

Any people depicted in stock imagery provided by Thinkstock are models, and such images are being used for illustrative purposes only. Certain stock imagery © Thinkstock.

Lulu Publishing Services rev. date: 8/1/2013

SimpleGuy Diet 2

SimpleGuy Diet 2

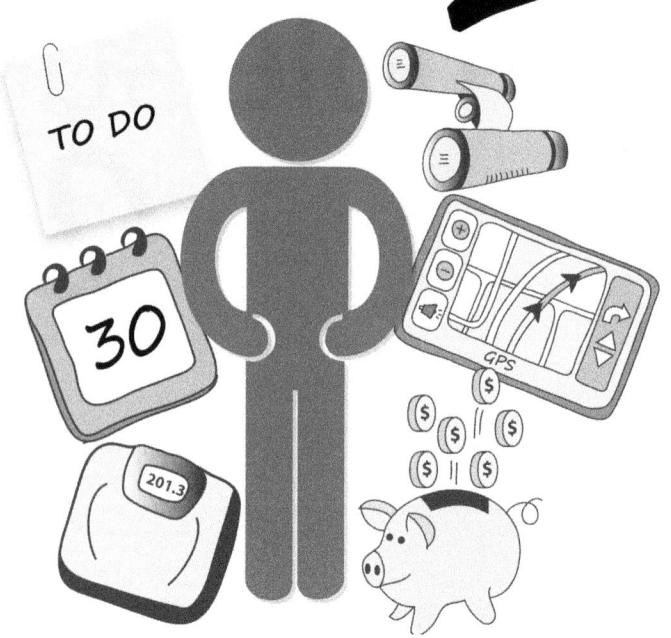

Dedication

This simple booklet is dedicated to you.
Congratulations on taking the first step towards better health and lowering the number on your bathroom scale by reading this simple booklet.
Enjoy!

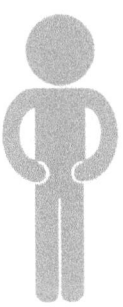

Welcome Back, My Brothers...

For those of you who read the original version of the Simple Guy Diet booklet, Welcome Back! This new version has all the goodness and honest simplicity of the first booklet... now with the addition of a couple of new chapters and some additional bonus insight. Although new and improved, it is as simple as ever...

Meet the Simple Guy

I am a pathetically average 50-something male. I have a job, a wife, two kids, a house and a small yard to mow. I weighed just under 180 pounds when I graduated college and, over time, I slowly worked my way up to 212. That works out to about a pound a year of gain. I have always been healthy and have no medical issues, again, just pathetically normal.

My wife is smarter, more disciplined and a better athlete than me. Last year, on her birthday, she decided to start a slight lifestyle change to lose a bit of weight. She forked over a small recurring monthly fee for some famous Internet diet program and immediately started to assign "points" to everything she consumed. She joined an online group and rallied some of her friends to start walking with her every day. This sounded crappy to me; everything she was doing sounded like work, and thus, I had no interest in mirroring her strategy.

In my small-minded way, I decided to focus on a couple super-simple food adjustments just to see what would happen. With virtually no effort in my first three months, I lost seven pounds. The next month I lost four more pounds and then three additional pounds fell off. No pills, no counting points, no gym membership, no equipment to buy—just simple self-managed changes. Now, after six months, I have taken about 20 pounds off of my starting weight and I'm in love with this low-effort process!

Many of my friends and co-workers ask me how this happened. They invite me to lunch or for a cup of coffee to have a little "one on one time" to extract the magic of my weight loss. What I have decided to do is spend some time to have a website created and populate it with simple information to better share my success. After thousands of visits to our website (www.simpleguydiet.com), I was urged to publish this booklet and have The Simple Guy Diet available to those who would prefer a paperback rather than a download. I have worked hard to keep the publishing/distribution costs as low as possible to deliver the best possible value for your hard-earned money.

Again, please enjoy the information and the adventure of this simple weight loss story. I know this is what worked for me... and, hopefully, it will work as a great place to start for you as well!

Just so we are 100% clear, I do not consider myself to be an "author", but rather, a storyteller... and... this is not a book, but a booklet. I have far too much respect for those who write as a profession to ever attempt to claim any of their hard earned turf. So... please find a comfortable place to sit and in about a half an hour you will know the path of my complete journey... and, hopefully, have some initial thoughts on how yours will begin. To get full value from this tiny booklet, grab a pen, circle some words, scribble in the margin or dog-ear the pages that hit home for you. This is YOUR booklet, so start now and put it to work for you!

My Inspiration

People often ask my why I created the Simple Guy Diet. It was part out of personal need, part sharing my success, part creating accessibility to friends and family and part based on inspiration from a couple of business books I read years ago.

Have you ever read the books FISH! (Stephen Lundin) or The One Minute Manager (Ken Blanchard)? They are wonderfully short, yet profoundly effective business-related books; one is about organizational development and the other is about general leadership. Neither will make you a specialist on either topic, but what each will do is share a story or two for you to adapt into your own world. Rather than "how-to," The One Minute Manager and FISH! focus on business situations that will hopefully inspire you to think differently and potentially find new solutions which lead to change. On a personal level, the style of each of these books really clicked for me...and I believe, to the millions of others who read them.

The "voice" and message of The Simple Guy Diet is somewhat the same. The Simple Guy Diet is a story of a real person, me, and my simplified approach to lowering the number on my bathroom scale. This is not a step by step "how to" diet book chock-a-block full of recipes, but rather, a "one guy to another" story respecting both your time and those precious greenbacks in your wallet.

This booklet is short by design... and contains no fluff or fillers. It is just my story and contains what I think you will need to know in order to get out of the gate and be successfully on your way to both lower weight and improved health. Please read every word, including the BLOG WISDOM at the end. That is the section where you will get a sense of my thoughts and emotions in the months and years after initially starting the Simple Guy Diet. Please enjoy this quick read and apply it to your own life and unique set of circumstances. With a small and focused commitment, you will be happily taking your first step to a healthier you!!

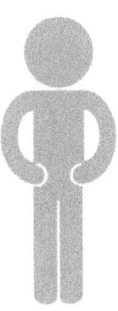

FYI, All Diets Are Great!

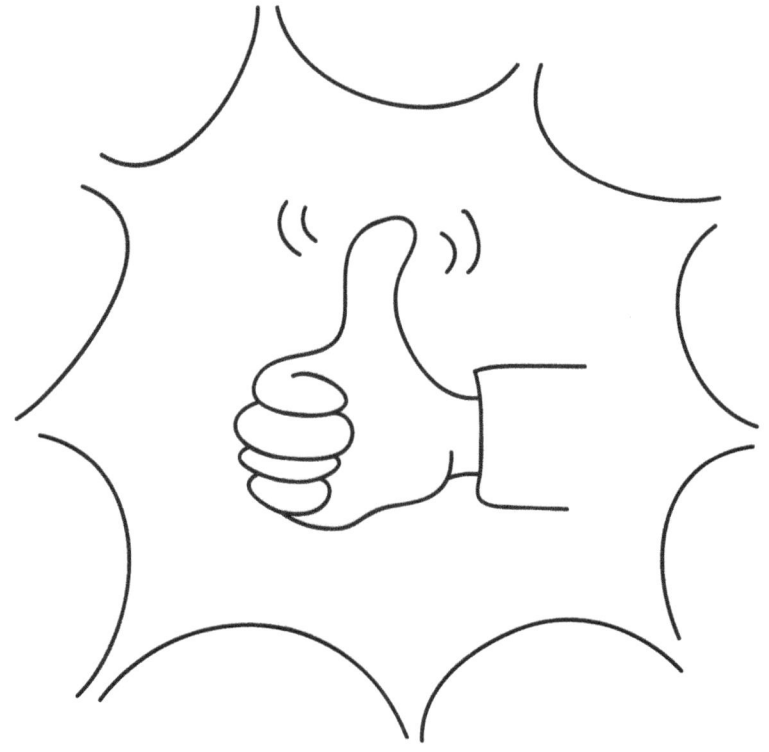

FYI, All Diets Are Great!

There are hundreds of diets out there... maybe even thousands!! Knowing YOU want to lose weight is great, but if you are anything like me, some of the biggest hurdles I faced were:

- Which diet is right for me?
- How much money am I willing to spend?
- What kind of life altering commitment am I willing to make?

Additional self-reflection challenged me on "what kind of dieter am I?" What would be the best approach for me to take in order to have the best shot at success? My options of pathways to follow were numerous, and was I to:

- Understand how my body works?
- Sign up with a national weight loss program?
- Buy a bottle of weight loss pills at my local grocery/drug store?
- Trust a celebrity endorser?
- Hire a personal trainer?
- Buy a juicer?

- Join an on-line group for support?

- Go it alone and start working out to sweat off the pounds?

Although each program claims to have excellent results, I just could not pull the trigger and select a single option. Over the years I tried a couple of different methods, all of which worked... at least for a while. Sooner or later, I fell off the wagon, and the pounds (which I had strategically melted away) seemed to creep back on. At some point, I think I found it easier to get myself to believe that maybe, just maybe, this was the size and the weight I was supposed to be. That emotion would feel good for a while, then the reality of how I looked, how I felt, how my clothes fit... and how I knew what I would like to be would cloud my "surrender to chubbiness" thinking.

Somehow I believed that there was a diet that was right for me... somewhere (likely, not dissimilar for singles looking for the perfect mate). The sea of options and opportunities to lose weight was so vast that I felt somewhere between lost and hopeless. Going to a bookstore (and we have some awesome ones in my town) would totally bum me out. I felt unqualified and almost vulnerable as each well thought, well written, diet book title was calling, "Pick me", "No, pick me" as I walked aimlessly up and down the diet isle.

The information certainly all exists, and certainly there is the perfect weight loss method for each and every one of us. I almost wanted someone to tell me what to do... find the right answer for me, as it was clear that I certainly did not know which way to turn.

I lived in "diet purgatory" for years, starting/trying one thing or another with my typical half-baked commitment. My results were predictable... lousy! As I mentioned in the introduction, my (awesome) wife decided to focus a bit on her personal weight loss. To be expected, she did all the right things to be successful by becoming educated and then selecting a plan...and sticking to it.

She prompted me to do the same, but with my years of failed attempts (and being honest with myself) I knew this would be just another sleigh ride to hell. I wisely resisted her invitation to partner up with her on her well-chosen method.

Personally, I think I (really) fail when I am "not sure", or not "all in".

Although the perfect diet or diet method (for me) certainly exists, I just couldn't cope with all the choices or even get motivated to sift through all the options. Stubborn-ass male thinking swiftly took over and I decided to shun the educated world of diet expertise and try it my own way. I am sure you can picture the guy building the IKEA bookshelves and ignoring the instructions... or the guy refusing to ask for directions. Sadly, that was me, now going down the diet road alone.

Looking back, I seemingly gave up on "following" and just decided to "lead"... to control my own destiny. Perhaps this was some weird form of me taking control... or perhaps a way of not failing, as I never really started anything... at least not formally. How can you fall off the wagon if you were never on it in the first place... right? Man, I love being a guy!

In retrospect (now having several years of living the Simple Guy method under my belt), this simple diet philosophy was the absolute right thing to do... for me. It ticked all of my critical boxes and allowed me to be in absolute control for very little cost and a marginal effort.

I will be the first person to say that all major diet programs are great... even excellent. What the Simple Guy approach will do, is get you started. It will allow you to prove to yourself that you can control your own destiny, that you can have success, and you can have a bit of fun while losing weight in your own managed way. Let's face it, our goals and our needs are all different based on our:

- age
- finances
- starting weight
- goals
- health
- abilities
- commitment level
- desire

Personally, one of the real keys to the kingdom is just "commitment". Again, starting with a "play fair" attitude for 30 days will serve as your best test... and a fantastic launching pad.

I truly believe that men and women have different thought processes around being committed (news flash!).

To that end, this is why the Simple Guy Diet is:

1. A great place to start and

2. A method that only requires a short span of time to test drive the concept

We all know what the end game looks like for most of the highly marketed diet plans… it is the guy holding a monstrous sized pair of jeans with the happy dieter, of half their starting size, smiling ear to ear. If that is your goal, then starting with the Simple Guy is just fine; however, you will definitely need additional professional help along the way. If you are ready to make the personal, financial and emotional commitment to a well-run national diet plan, I say, "Go for it"… as you are certainly ahead of me!! But, if you are a bit lost (maybe I still am), I whole-heartedly suggest you give the Simple Guy Diet a try. Your investment in time, energy and money will be very, very small and solely managed by you. Once you see how easy it is to lose a bit of weight and manage your own road to success; then, perhaps you can investigate taking the next step to a larger, more structured diet plan. Before you get married to a higher cost, higher commitment program, please use the Simple Guy philosophy as your "engagement" to dieting. I would think that if you do graduate to a well-run national diet method, your odds of success would be heightened with a jump-start to your confidence via the Simple Guy Diet.

Some people like to jump in the pool… for me, I am more comfortable wading in… just to make sure. For me, the Simple Guy Diet was enough to accomplish what I had started out to do... lose 20 pounds. For others, it will be merely a great place to start... a test drive if you will, in successful dieting. I strongly urge you to continue to check out as many diets as possible so you can find the one that is best for you. The real goal is for YOU finding YOUR best way to manage your weight... not who can sell the most books or generate the most revenue.

I think there is something profoundly wonderful how all of us learned to walk before we ever ran. The Simple Guy Diet will serve as a pleasurable dieting walk... so lace up and get ready to rumble towards better health.

The following "chapterettes" are very, very short by design. This plan is NOT complicated... then again, how could it be... it's from me. Please enjoy and remember to read cover to cover. Thanks!

My To-Do List

✔ Commit to 30 days (the hardest part!)

✔ Buy a digital scale

✔ Have a food road map

✔ Celebrate your inner-cheapness

✔ Enjoy the view

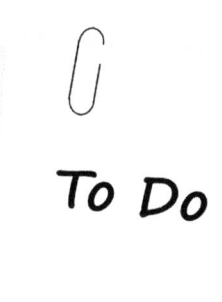

Commit to 30 Days

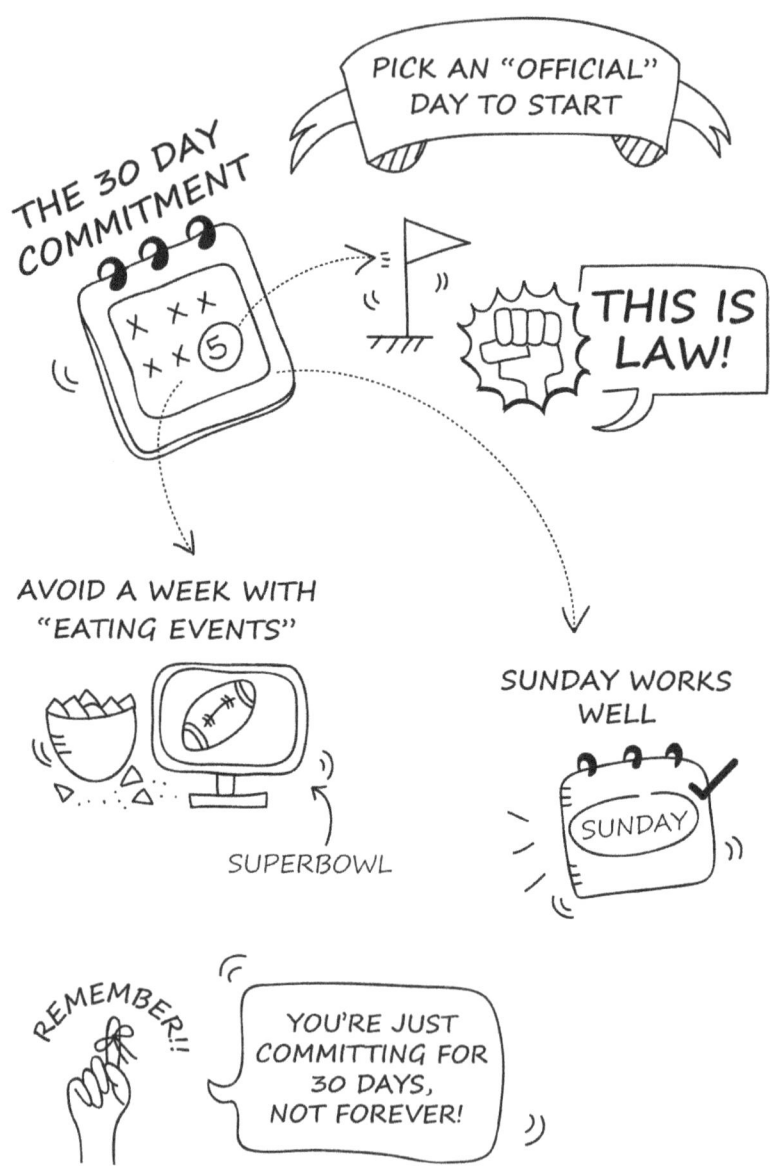

Commit to 30 Days

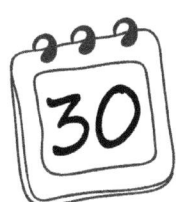

Before you do anything, you need to select an official day to start and declare it as law! To give yourself the best chance at success, try to start where you have no big "eating" events in the first couple of weeks like the Super Bowl, an office party or your neighborhood block party. I found it best to start on a Sunday so you can control what you do the day before falling into your soon to change workweek routine. Remember, you are not changing forever, just for 30 days to see if this adjustment fits your lifestyle. Once you get to your 30-day anniversary, then, if you have been successful, it is your choice to continue. I started with 30 days and have not stopped. In fact, it just gets easier and more empowering!

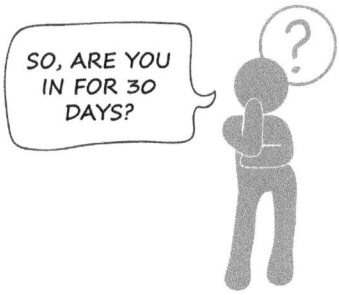

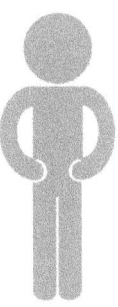

Buy a Digital Scale

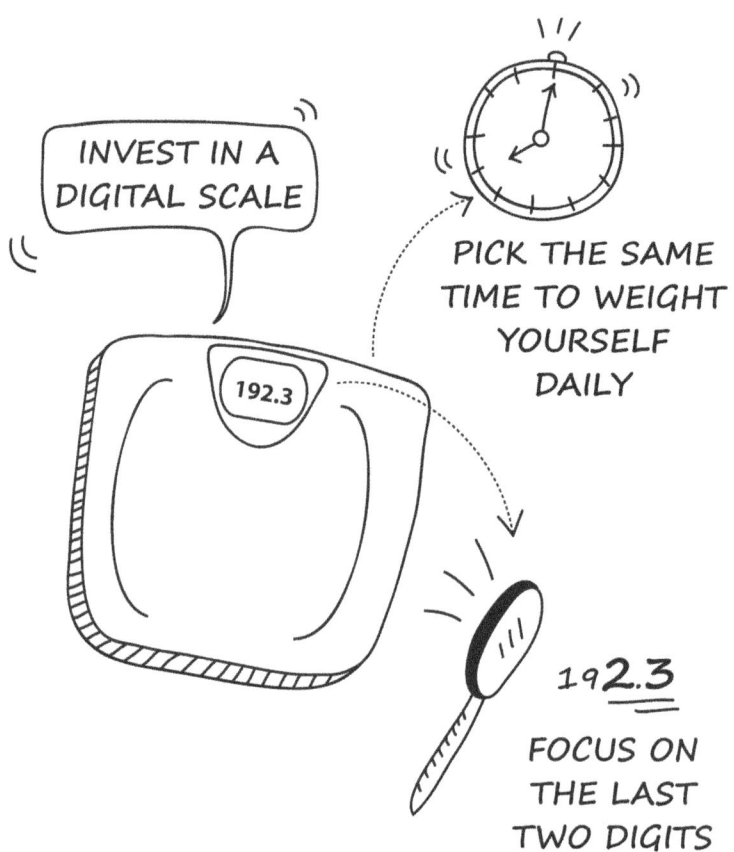

Buy a Digital Scale

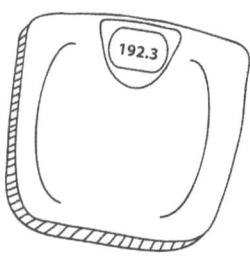

Rather than spending money on pills, special foods or online programs, I strongly suggest that the first thing you do is go to your local store, department store, on-line retailer, Walmart or Target and buy a DIGITAL scale. You really need to have a scale before your first day. This will start you on the road to honesty. My wife is a big believer in the scale and hops on it every morning. For the first month, I weighed myself once a week, every Monday morning before I took my shower. It is important that you find a time to serve as your "baseline weigh-in time". Your weight naturally fluctuates during the course of the day, so pick a time that works best for you and weigh-in the same time and same day of the week for your first four weeks. After your first month, I would recommend that you weigh yourself every day (at the same time each day).

The great part of a digital scale is that it is brutally accurate. This little devise should be considered to be your new best friend or your new worst enemy depending on how things are going. After my initial month of weight loss, which was seven pounds for me, I started to focus on the last two digits of the scale for my morning, pre-shower, weigh in. As an example: If the scale read 196.4, I would tell myself "64," representing the last two digits. The next day I might be "62" and in several days "54." I found this to be both rewarding and motivating by just focusing on the last two numbers. This way, every little change, even a tenth of a pound, felt like a personal victory—and a great reason to stick to the plan.

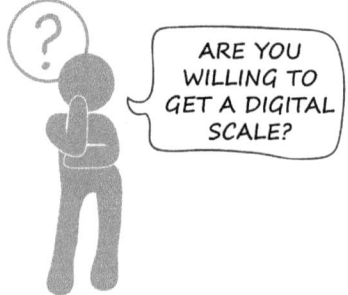

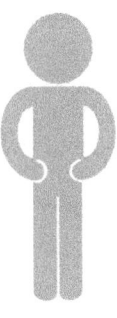

My Food Road Map

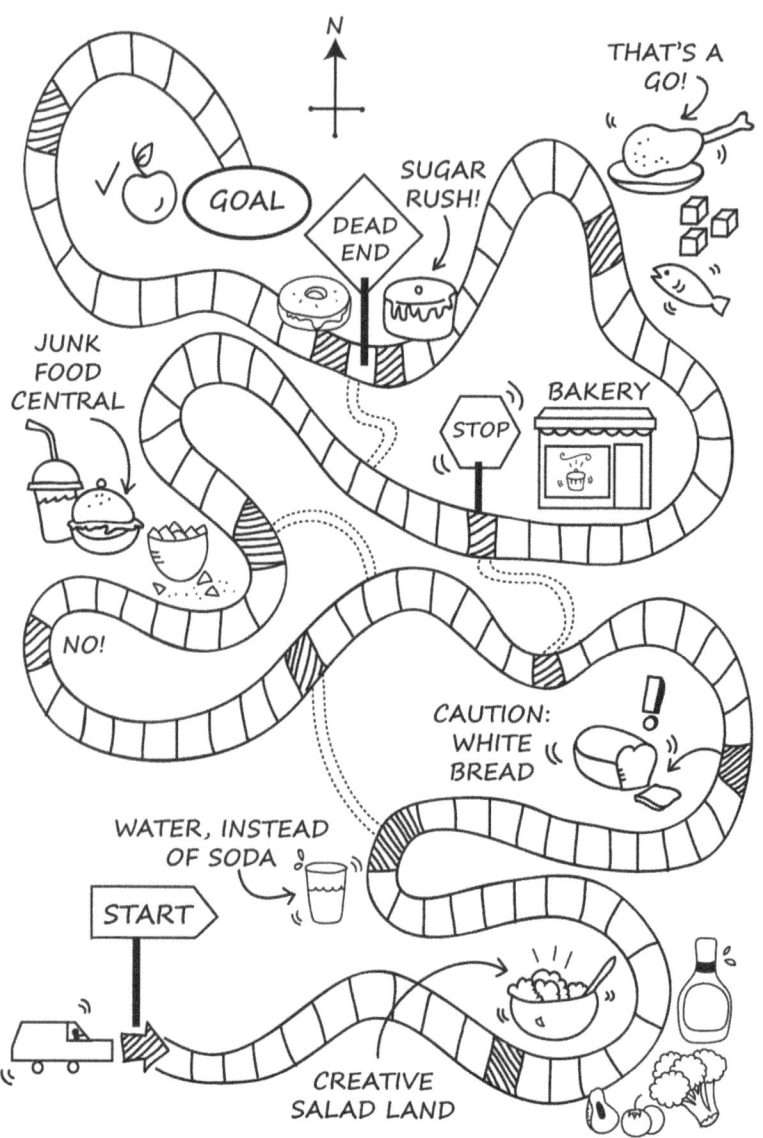

My Food Road Map

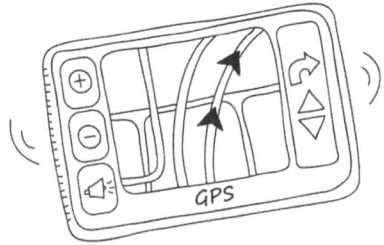

As I refuse to have things be difficult, I chose a logical and unscientific approach... as I am both logical and unscientific.

I eliminated "obvious carbs" from my diet. From my very first day, I gave up all bread, rice, potatoes and tortillas (and I love tortillas!). I certainly was NOT carb free. I continued to eat my bowl of instant oatmeal with a handful of Post grape-nuts, a palm full of crushed walnuts and a quarterish-cup of 1% milk as I had always had for breakfast. I also eliminated most desserts for the first month. When I need a sweet fix, I do occasionally have a cut up apple sprinkled with cinnamon and sugar, a small coffee mug full of regular vanilla yogurt and grape-nuts, or some small pieces of refrigerated dark chocolate as my evening dessert.

OK, deep breath. If you are in, you're in! Although these changes are simple and somewhat obvious, you really need to embrace these adjustments for 30 days. If you are wearing your "I don't want to pants", or your "all diets stink pants" or even your very unattractive "bitchy pants", you will need to take those bad-boys off and replace them with your favorite "I'll give it a try pants". Part of the change will need to be attitude... so make these changes fun and accept them as a challenge rather than an obstacle.

Some Random Tips:

- If it is white, don't eat it (bread, rice, potatoes, tortillas, etc.)

- Eliminate most soft drinks and replace with water (I added a pinch of Crystal Light lemonade powder for a little flavor. At home or at a self-serve restaurant, I filled my cup with 90% water and added a one second shot of Sprite or lemon-aid)

- Adios to french fries, adios to onion rings and adios to anything that is cooked in a fryer

- Keep a pack of gum in your car, a pack next to your TV, one more at work and/or any other place you typically want to snack. Sometimes keeping your mouth occupied with gum can prevent unneeded and usually evil snacking

- Find things that are not bad for you to fall in love with (for me it was a tall americano at Starbucks)

- For the first 30 days, just say no to desserts, doughnuts (I love doughnuts even more than I do tortillas) and anything in a bakery case

- Remember, the first bite of anything is always the best. So if you are going to have dessert, just have one bite of someone else's

Again, this shift in eating will seem a bit odd at first. I remember thinking to myself, "How can I make a stinkin' sandwich without any bread?" You will soon see that our wonderful society of on the go eating requires some kind of "carby vessel" like bread slices, a tortilla or a hamburger bun to hold in the contents. You will quickly learn that all the good stuff tends to live inside the bread and the bun. So continue to eat the good stuff and ditch "the container" (the bread) which is little more than a distraction to nutrition and a boost to your waistline.

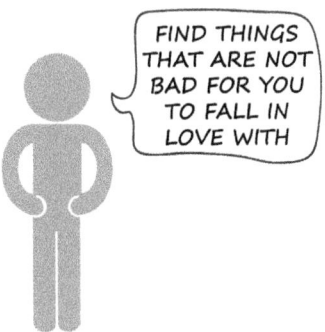

THINGS THAT HAPPENED TO ME:

- I craved crunchy!! I loved having a half dozen baby carrots or a handful of raw almonds for a snack; almonds are great for the office too

- For some weird reason, I had a coffee mug full of red wine most evenings, but just one

- For the first time in my life, I ate dark chocolate (at least 70% cocoa); I would have a piece the size of two to four postage stamps (also, keep it in the fridge, it's a million times better)

- I really started focusing on my personal, no evil indulgence everyday. My tall americano was always a welcome highlight… a couple of times a day

- Although it took a bit of time, I really craved consistency in what I was eating… rather than always searching for new and different

- Who knew water could be a beverage? It has become my go-to fluid and I am loving it hot, cold or warm

LUNCH IDEAS:

Since I work for a pretty big company, many times I do not have the time for a full hour to eat or had convenient access to our cafeteria depending on my building assignment. Coupled with the fact that packing my own lunch was not a good option (too unfun) for me, the following worked (when I first started):

1.) Go to McDonalds and order a side salad and a McDouble (each off the dollar menu) and a cup of water. Use no more than 25% of the dressing packet, put the lid back on and shake it up. As for the McDouble, take the top and the bottom bun off and move it aside. With what is left, take the plastic knife from the salad kit and cut the burger into multiple pieces, making it last a bit longer. I hate to admit this, but (pre-Simple Guy Diet) I went to McDonalds a couple of times a week, so I had to find how to make this old and sadly familiar habit fit into a diet regimen. Try to modify some of your favorites, so you aren't feeling too restricted in your new lifestyle. There was something strangely comfortable about eating at McDonalds for me. I am not sure if it was the familiarity of the colors, the ease of the menu, carrying the tray or the quick service. In my heart of hearts, I know this is not the best food choice for me; but there was something "very right" for me to keep coming back. If you do gravitate to some of your favorite spots, try and understand why you are there and then make a big effort to modify what you consume to stay on the plan.

2.) If you happen to have a Costco or grocery store nearby, purchase the pre-made chicken Caesar salad. Ditch the croutons and use no more than half of the salad dressing offered. Again, place the lid back on, and while holding the lid, shake it like crazy to get it all mixed up. Eat half and save the other half for your lunch the next day. Be sure to keep the plastic fork in the container, as finding a replacement fork the next day can be problematic. Hopefully you have a fridge at work to store your food treasure for the next day.

3.) If you are a "brown-bagger", be sure that two things happen:

- Keep it as carb-free as possible and

- Pack things you like and look forward to consuming. This will allow you to become the master of your own happiness!

4.) What really worked great for me, was to pop into a grocery store and buy 2 big 'ol Bugs Bunny carrots and an apple of my choice. I always had water available at work, so I was good to go. I was very surprised what a good, fast and satisfying lunch this was for me.

DINNER IDEAS:

1.) Personally, I have had great success with buying bags or pre-washed plastic tubs of salad at my local grocery store. Do not buy the ones with dressing in the bag, as many times these are packaged with other evil things... like wonton sticks in the oriental salad. Add different veggies you may have on hand to maintain variety and that all-important CRUNCH. I use a squirt of Hidden Valley Ranch Dressing and a generous amount of black pepper. Most weeks I buy a pre-cooked baked rotisserie chicken at the grocery store and cut up a piece to mix in with my salad

2.) I try to find some kind of meat or fish as my main entree (rather than a monster salad as my main dish) once or twice a week. When I do, my evening glass of red wine seems to get consumed for dinner (again, you only get one!). Add a side of steamed veggies or a small salad and you're good to go! I learned (from my wife) to really slow down and stretch out the time it takes to consume the meal, excellent advice indeed! If buying a pre-made chicken or barbecuing meat isn't happening, then a lightly doctored up can of tuna will also be a good time saving, easy to prepare trick

3.) Bad news, my brothers, steer clear of beer

4.) As a salad was my main dinner item, I was sure to add different veggies to build in plenty of variety (more on this in the pages to come)

5.) If you need more volume to eat when you start out, just add more lettuce to your master bowl... in fact, knock your socks off! Lettuce is good... but beware... the dressing you add is likely NOT your dietary friend, so think before you pour

6.) Attempt to get to the point where your "base ingredients" and your portions become somewhat automatic. For me, a handful of mixed greens, a cupped hand of slaw mix, and a cupped handful of shredded carrots. This equation seems to get me to 90% of what I need for dinner. The simpler you can make it, the better

7.) When I go eat out for dinner with my family or for business I try and stick to a game plan. First of all, I try and have an idea what I am going to order before I even sit down. I come in with good intentions to order a salad and then somehow I panic and order the chicken quesadilla when the server shows up. Stay focused on the small stuff (starters and sides) and this will be life changing! I typically order a small house salad and a side of hot veggies. I have totally given up at even looking at entrees for a couple of reasons... the portions are too darn big and it is typically a bad value. Turn the tables on "feeling bad about eating less" and spin the thinking in to "permission to save money" when you go out to eat!

Simple Guy Diet 2

DON'T FORGET DESSERT:

#1 A cut up apple sprinkled with cinnamon & sugar

#2 A small piece of dark chocolate (stored in the fridge)

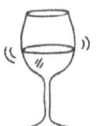

#3 A small coffee mug (portion) of wine... assuming you are of legal drinking age!

#4 A small coffee mug with yogurt and grape-nuts

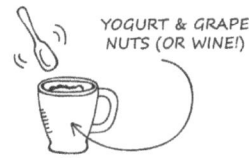

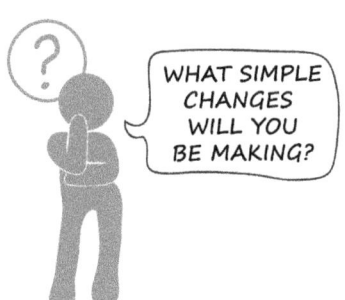

The Simple Guy's Dining Out Favorites

<u>Old Problem</u>   <u>New Solution</u>

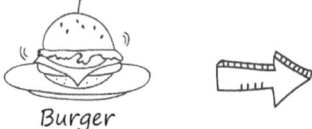
Burger

Lose the bun, lose the mayo and wrap that burger in lettuce. My local McDonald's, In-N-Out, Burger King and Five Guys are all happy to sell you the burger of your choice without the bun.

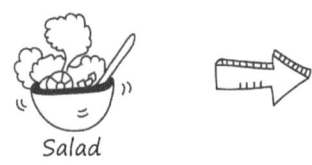
Salad

Ditch the croutons and ask for the dressing on the side (using no more than half of the dressing!) I also take the first bite before adding the dressing.

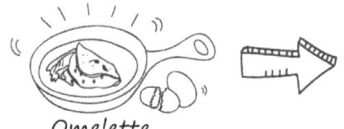
Omelette

An excellent choice is an omelette, but get it al a carte, without the toast or the hash browns. This will be good for ANY meal of the day... in any country

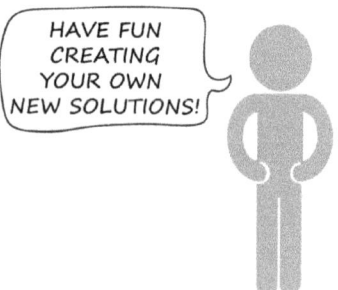

HAVE FUN CREATING YOUR OWN NEW SOLUTIONS!

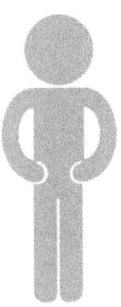

Be the Genius Salad Maker You Know You Are

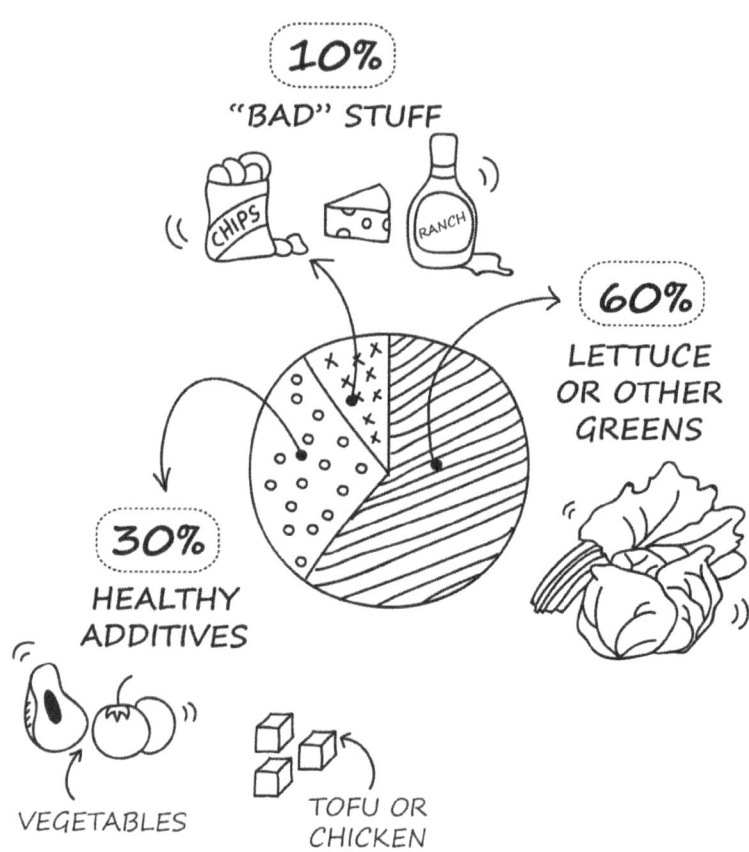

Be the Genius Salad Maker You Know You Are

Nobody knows what you like more than you!! Now, the goal is how to create the ultimate win-win food; a salad that is "look-forward-to-good" and still allows you to work toward your weight reduction goal. Below are some good things to think about before you dive in. Hopefully, these tips will get you started on your pathway to salad preparation success.

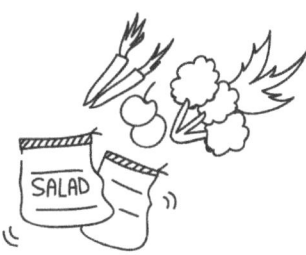

SALAD MAKING TIPS:

- Clean out your fridge of foods you no longer need as these are just distractions

- Purchase two or three of your favorite dressings (I have two)

- Dedicate yourself to become the best salad maker you know

- Find ways to treat yourself with salad "additives"

- Don't be afraid to add things that you never had in a salad before

- Find a "master bowl" to call your own… and use the same one each night for dinner (for me, I have a bowl that is capable of holding six cups of water). My salads only fills about half the bowl, the extra room makes it ideal to mix up without creating a major mess

- Use a different beverage on different nights to help add variety to your daily masterpiece

- Purchasing bags or plastic tubs of lettuce in your local grocery store is a great way to simplify and find plenty of variety with your cornerstone ingredient

- Rule the vegetable aisle; be sure to have plenty of other veggies on hand to mix in, and when you know things are not healthy add-ins, play fair

- Be daring! If your salads are feeling a bit bland, squirt a tablespoon full of BBQ sauce or sweet Thai chili (in addition to salad dressing) can really become a game changer

- Find your cornerstone ingredients; be sure to always have them on hand in your fridge. For me, store pre-packaged mixed greens, a bag of shredded slaw mix and a bag of shredded carrots are always in plentiful supply in my fridge

In addition to the above where you can have endless options, here are a couple of my "no-miss" favorite dinner salads when I am not feeling too creative (read: lazy):

Simple Guy Diet 2

THE 60-30-10 PLAN:

I have found this to be a good working proportion in my salad making creations. I have 60% of my bowl contents be lettuce + (lettuce from a head or from a store bought bag/container), 30% will be what I call "healthy additives" (like the shredded carrots and slaw mix) and 10% "bad stuff". Below is an expanded explanation to give you a better idea of each ingredient category:

Lettuce + (60%)

- Pre-packaged (a generous hand scoop equals about one serving)

- Whole head (about 1/4 head equals one serving)

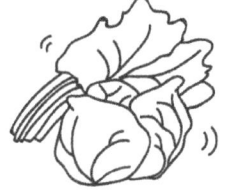

- Shredded slaw mix (pre-packaged near the lettuce... and darn cheap)

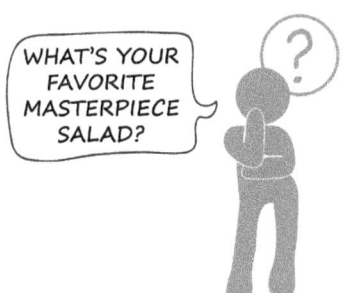

Healthy Additives (30%)

- A palm full of shelled sunflower seeds
- A palm full of chopped nuts
- Baby carrots / shredded carrots
- Freshly chopped veggies
- Grilled veggies
- Spiced up tofu
- Lean meat or fish of your choice (4 ounces)
- Ground pepper
- Avocado
- Chopped fresh fruit
- Salsa

Bad Stuff (10%)

- Salad Dressing (one heaping tablespoon)
- Ice cream scoop size of tuna or chicken salad
- Palm full (4 to 6 chips) of crunched up Ruffles potato chips… regular or BBQ (really!)

Simple Guy Diet 2

- Croutons (palm full)... this is an occasional treat

- A palm full of shredded cheese

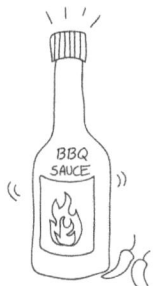

- Sauce It Up!! Since we just touched on "bad stuff", here is another bad stuff variety idea that has worked well for me. Try adding a tablespoon of your favorite flavor craving sauce in to your salad. I seem to always start with a little squirt of ranch dressing; then, on some days, I add a tablespoon of BBQ sauce or sweet Thai chili sauce. Each of these additives (the ranch, the BBQ and the sweet Thai chili) are all calorie and nutritional nightmares. The way I see it, an occasional "tablespoon of this or that" is a heck of a lot better for you eating a store-bought frozen chicken pot pie or knocking down several slices of pizza for dinner.

- Remember to use the "bad stuff" sparingly and please try and play fair for the first 30 days

One of the questions I receive is, "What is your favorite masterpiece salad?" About once a week I really go for it and make what I believe to be is my ultimate salad, which I affectionately refer to as my "Heaven and Hell Salad." Although the ingredients vary from week to week, it may contain the following:

- 1/2 of a medium sized avocado

- Six BBQ Ruffle potato chips, crushed up

- One heaping tablespoon of ranch dressing

- 1/3 bag of store bought heart of romaine lettuce (in my "master bowl")

- A palm full of shelled sunflower seeds

- Two tablespoons of medium ground pepper (that's a ton... but I love it!)

- A palm full of cut up chicken

- 1/3 of a cucumber, diced

- 6 baby carrots

- 6 baby tomatoes cut in half

I realize my masterpiece may not be for everyone, but certainly you will identify your own dinner work of art. Remember, to keep variety in what you make. If you are anything like me, you will have a couple of "go to" salads which always do the trick. At first, the building and the creation part is what I liked least... but now, it is absolutely my favorite part and I feel I am the king of the veggie aisle at my local grocery store... and, my brothers, it's good to be king!

Another one of my favorite salads to make the one I call my "Magic Layer Salad". This bad-boy is super simple and seems to make me happy every time I make it... in fact, this one was for quite a while, my daily "go to" salad.

- handful of store bought mixed greens (on a plate, rather than a bowl)

- a bed to of slaw mix to cover the greens
- sprinkle shredded carrots on to the top of the slaw mix
- a palm-full of diced red onions
- a palm-full of (shelled) sunflower seeds
- a couple tablespoons of olive oil and a couple of tablespoons of balsamic vinegar
- a half of a diced up avocado if they are in season, let it sit in the fridge for 5-10 minutes, then enjoy!!

Some days I am not that hungry and I feel like using a big boy plate rather than my bowl. I start with a salad size plate, then I create a small bed (covering most of the plate) of either mixed greens or slaw mix. Slice up a whole tomato or cut in half 6-10 cherry tomatoes, use half an avocado (either sliced or cubed) applying to lettuce/slaw bed. Since this is a smaller portion, I take four Wheat Thin crackers and divide a little block of single serving cheddar cheese (.75 ounce size from the deli area in your grocery store), divide the cheese into quarters and place a piece on each Wheat Thin to create a fantastic mini-meal. Be sure to try this one with your small glass of red wine!

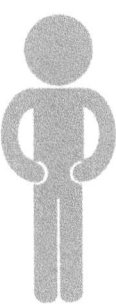

Celebrate Your Inner Cheapness

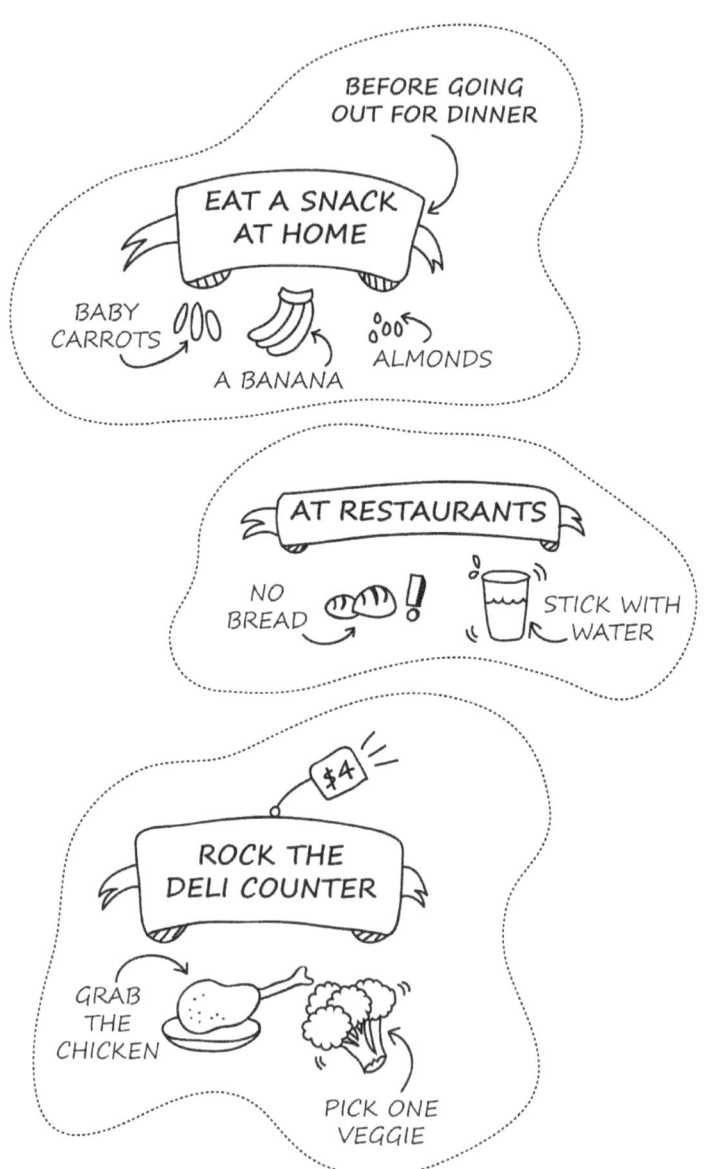

Celebrate Your Inner Cheapness

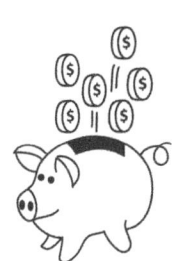

For me, the joy of spending less money was almost as fun as watching the pounds melt away. Not purchasing bread items, desserts, beer, chips and processed snacks clearly was a money saver. Discovering low carb ways to eat off the dollar menu and living without soda was a huge eye opener. Things like baby carrots and buying a prepackaged whole cooked chicken at the local grocery store will highlight what great values there are when you eat in a sensible, low-carb way. I now find myself shopping less in the middle of the grocery store and now have the majority of my little shopping basket coming from the fruit and veggie section… OK, the red wine section too.

Here's a good idea if you and your family are going out to eat, have a small self-managed snack (either 10 baby carrots, a banana, or handful of almonds) while you are waiting for your team to saddle up before you go out. Then, at the restaurant, drink only water (or iced tea or coffee if you want to go a bit crazy financially) and have the house salad. As I mentioned earlier in the book, it is good to have a food strategy BEFORE you go in to dine. I typically do not look at the menu. As the more I look, the more I can talk myself into eating something less than good for me. I start to cook up excuses why it might be OK to order the chili cheeseburger. Bad rationale like, "I would never make

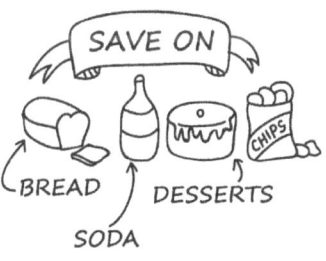

this for myself at home", or "Live it up, I'm eating out tonight" or "It's just one meal". Trust me, before you fall off the wagon, try and stay ON the wagon for at least 30 days. Also, beware of the bread or other goodies they put on the table prior to the arrival of your food. In the words of my Italian friend, Guido, "No bread!" This is the key to the kingdom... and a most evil table temptation! What you will quickly see, as I have, is how much you spend when you eat out for things that aren't at all beneficial to you... and your weight loss strategy. Eating consciously, more fresh and in a low-carb manner will save you a ton of money!

Also, a good food source for those daily lunches or simple take home evening meals, is in a full service grocery store with a deli counter. Most of the larger regional and national grocery chain stores offer various premade options. As an example, for a lunch, I would set a budget of $4. Then I would choose from the deli counter, eliminating anything that has been fried. No orange chicken, no egg rolls, no corn dogs and avoid anything with big carbs like potato salad and pasta salad. Be sure one of the items is veggie-based. If you do get a bit lost in all the options, a couple of slices of lean meat and a single slice of cheese is an awesome place to start. I have found this to be a great way to get a big and adventurous bang for my buck and it is an awesome trick for any meal as well!

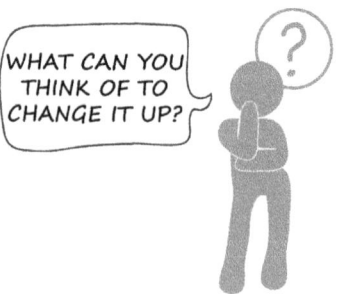

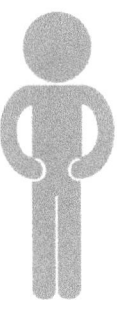

Enjoy the View

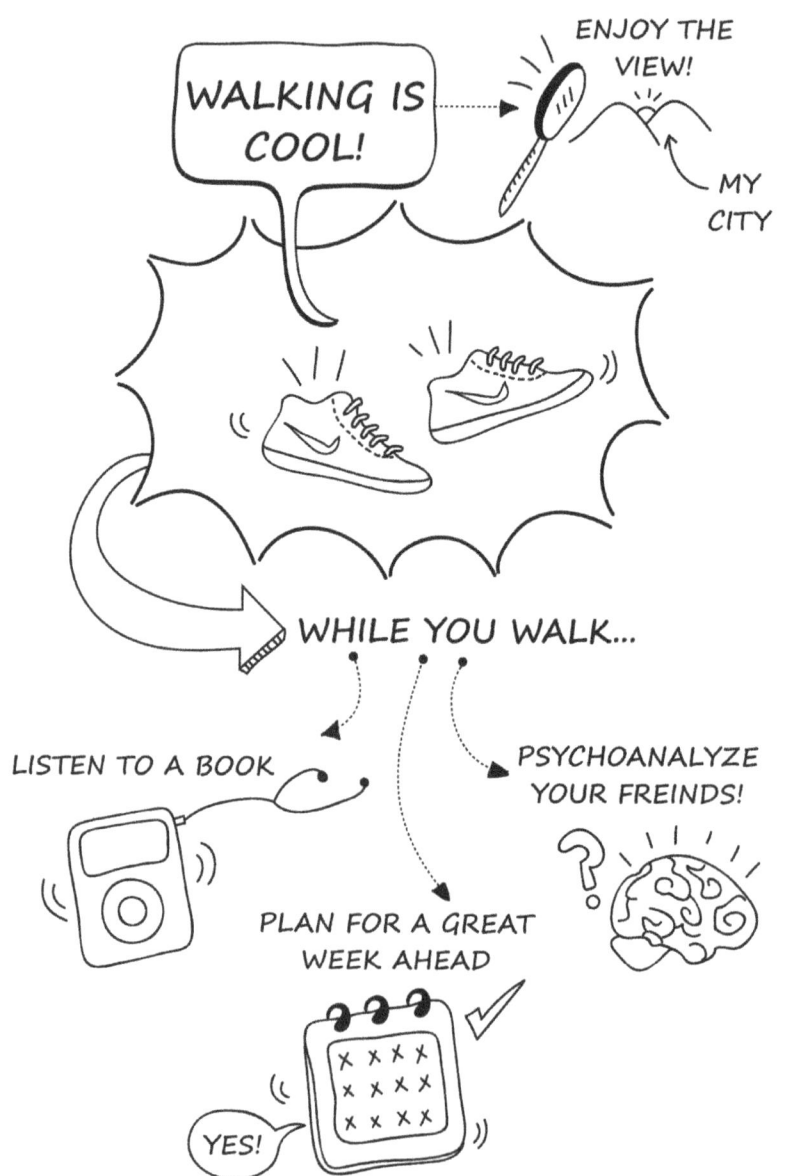

Enjoy the View

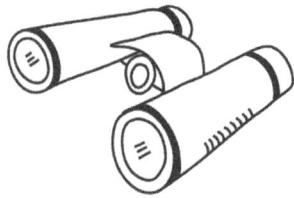

I was an athlete in high school and athletic in college. Sports had always been an important part of my life. Sometime in my mid-40s, the weekly basketball pick-up games stopped, I lost all interest in running in organized events, my gym membership (which I still have) has become little more than a recurring monthly bill and no longer did I have much interest in playing tennis.

I still very much love all of these activities, but rarely do them... and if/when I do, it is not with any regularity. Somehow, I am now more concerned about avoiding injury than I am about being physically active or competitive. It sounds weird, but it is true.

My wife, as I mentioned earlier, started walking... big time. On the weekends she would walk me like a dog!! At first I scoffed at this, as it is not a sport and it certainly is not athletic. I have now grown to love our long, cruising around weekend walks—no matter what the weather. There is no equipment necessary (other than your favorite pair of Nikes) or team to join. Best of all, excuses not to do it are out the window! Fitness aside, I have also found this a great time to get caught up on last week's events, as well as get clear on what's cooking for next week with my wife or, if you go it alone, a super time to work through issues or just to think creatively. On many levels, walking has been a huge game changer for me both physically and emotionally!

I can't believe I'm saying this, but walking is cool. By hoofing it around I am seeing my local world in a whole new way... and just enjoying the view.

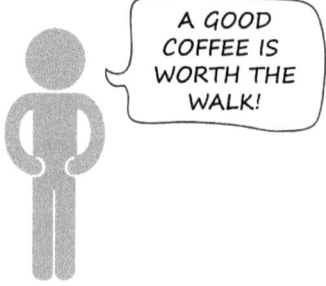

SYNERGIZE YOUR NEEDS (MULTI-TASK!) WHILE BEING ACTIVE

1.) Download and listen to a book while walking

2.) Make yard work part of your scheduled workout

3.) Assign yourself physical chores

4.) Do some physical activities with the kids

5.) Think about the day/week ahead while walking

6.) Wash your car by hand, just like your dad did

7.) The stairs are your friend... visit them often

8.) Walk a mile or two to your favorite coffee place

9.) Mentally align yourself for a great week at work

and my personal favorite...

10.) Psychoanalyze your friends and family members

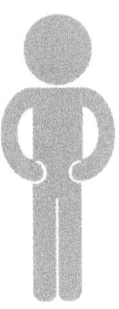

We All Stumble …

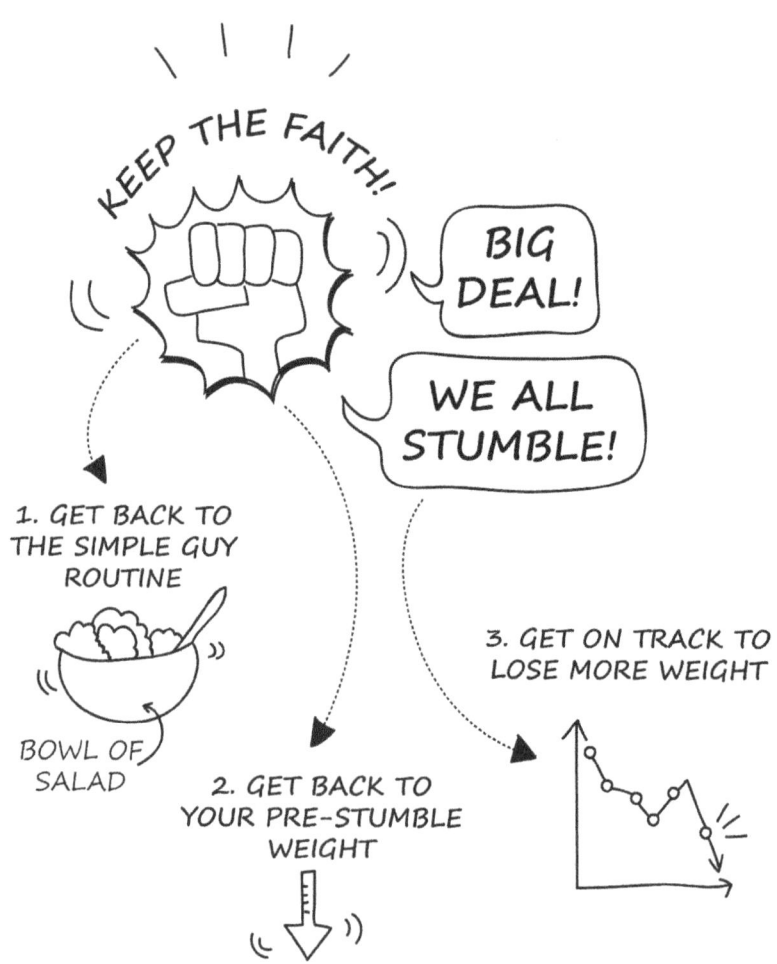

We All Stumble …

Worry not, Simple Guys, as we all stumble a bit from time to time, it's "a guy thing!"

Although you will be enjoying the fruits of your success as the pounds fall off with your new eating game plan, you will have small bursts of time when your weight is going the wrong way.

The good news (about the bad news) is that you will know why your scale is creeping northbound. There has likely been a "situation / event" which has taken you off your Simple Guy game. It just happens. The school reunion, a wedding weekend packed with activities, a family vacation, an extended birthday / anniversary celebration or a multi-day off-site meeting / conference for work are, for me, just plain bad.

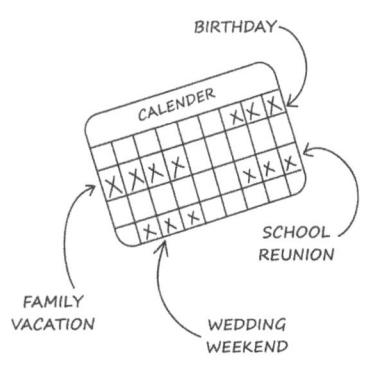

I have found that a multi-hour one-day event like a neighborhood block party, a football game watch party or an evening out with friends is totally manageable and only a little "slippage" may occur. But once I get into the multiday events, I really seem to fall back to my ways of old, even when I think I am managing them! Snacks, treats, chips and salsa seem to not only appear, but be calling my name. Even though I am conscious of what I am eating (which may be a victory by itself), I still onboard much more than I would when I am controlling my own routine.

I have learned that when I am out of my "controlled environment", I eat differently and ultimately gain a few pounds—to which I say, "Big deal!" The silver lining is that I now know that once I get back into my successful Simple Guy routine, in about a week (not a day or two), I will be back to my pre-vacation weight and right on track to slowly and sensibly lose more.

Keep the faith, my brothers, and happily know that the bumps in the road can be easily smoothed out.

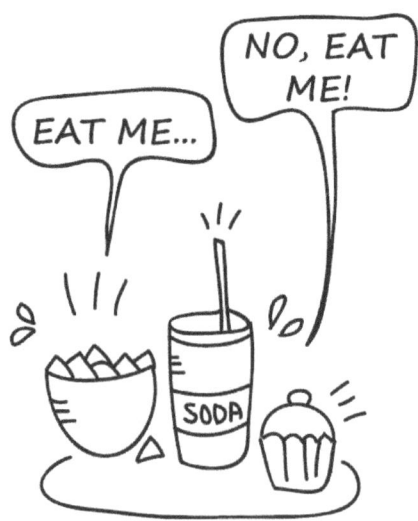

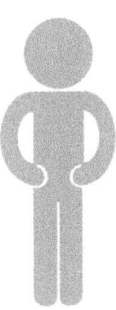

I Changed More Than My Weight

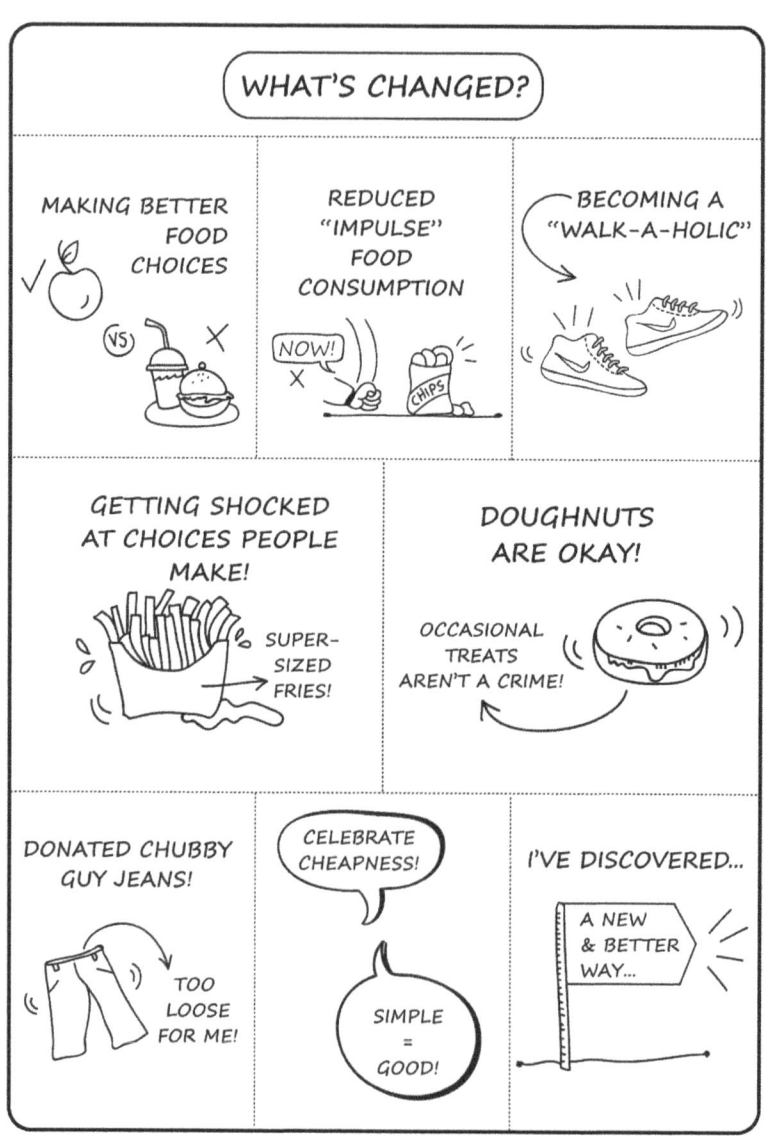

I Changed More Than My Weight

It's official... at least in my mind... that change has indeed occurred! Certainly I have dropped at least one jeans/pant size and my weight loss is now seemingly visible to all who know me. Here are several call outs of BIG things, which happened as the result of dropping some pounds over the first six months:

1.) I am not as interested in impulse food consumption as I was in the past.

2.) I am making better food choices and it seems absolutely natural to me.

3.) I am shocked when I watch others eat (by choice and quantity) and can't believe that was once me!

4.) I gave away a bunch of jeans and pants to Goodwill. Before this experience, I was always too cheap to give them away as I might need them again.

5.) I feel as if I am not compromising with my food intake; rather, I'm just living in a new and better way.

6.) I learned that losing weight, for me, was not about the food or the number on a scale. It was more about understanding my "triggers," like celebrating my inner cheapness, keeping it simple and NOT being told what to do that made this work for me.

7.) I love doughnuts! Although I did not have a doughnut for the first couple of months, when I did have one, it was absolutely awesome! Treating yourself every now and then is not a crime.

8.) I am thrilled with being a "junior walk-a-holic," as somehow in the past couple of years, physical activity got put on the back burner. Even though I am not working up a great sweat by walking, I love every step I take.

9.) I now know that I could indeed lose even more weight by increasing my exercise habits, adjusting my food once again, or by joining a more formalized program with professional guidance. At this point I am pretty darn happy where I am, and after six months, I am down about 20 pounds and still creeping down bit by bit.

Please remember, this is not a prescription or a guarantee. It is just something that worked very well for me. It is always a good idea to check in with your doctor before doing anything different. I wish you all the success in the world. Please have fun doing this for 30 days (and play fair) and see where it leads you. Everyone is different and being successful needs to be absolutely unique to you.

Do it for yourself... change is good!!!

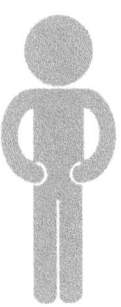

Six Easy Tips To Help You Get Started

Six Easy Tips To Help You Get Started

Once I started on the Simple Guy Diet, and then for the first year I started to find "little things" which seemed to really help me. Certainly you will find you own magic operating formula, but I thought it would be great to share several of my "greatest hits" with you!

1.) If you are attending a party, going to a bar or just having a lazy evening around the house and plan to have an indulgent drink or two, try and implement the Simple Guy "One—Two Punch". For every single serving of a calorie filled beverage you have (a glass of wine a full-strength soda), have two zero calorie beverages as your next two drinks. I have found this especially helpful if I attend a party. There is nothing worse that putting down your glass or continually saying, "No thanks" with your empty glass in hand. So keep your glass full and just manage what is in it… it's magic

2.) Before you saddle up to go out to eat with friends or family, be sure to grab a handful of baby carrots or raw almonds. This little snack will save you from showing up hungry and better allow you to stay on strategy. Walking in to a restaurant or your neighbor's backyard BBQ after having a little snack will better keep you in control to make the best choices possible

3.) Downsize your plates and bowls! When at home, try and replace the use of a dinner plate with a salad plate and a soup bowl with a smaller fruit bowl. There is something REALLY

GOOD about filling up a plate or bowl… so fill 'er up… just use a smaller one and I think you will soon see that there is equal satisfaction from a (smaller portion) plateful of food

4.) Your weight loss is all about you!! Try and keep things systematic and organized the way YOU want and this will be a great advantage. For me, I decided what I was going to eat and my desired portion size, then I tuned out all the clutter. Focusing on "your plan", rather than "all of the available options" will make a huge difference in your success. Find your own goodness and disregard all of the evil

5.) When you eat out… forget the entrée side of the menu even exists! What a huge game-changer this was for me. I usually order a small house salad and then one hot side order. Personally, I usually find some veggie thing, but if you really feel like you needed to consume something not so healthy, then pick a small side order in addition to your house salad. This will not only keep you better on track, but will also be a happy surprise to your wallet as well

6.) Find yourself a "master bowl"!! Find a bowl in your house, or go buy one that can be your salad portion control devise. For me, my bowl would hold six cups of water. When I make my daily dinner salad, my bowl is only about half full (although it was nearly full when I first started). Now, even after several years, I still use the same bowl nearly every night… creepy

Simple Guy BLOG Wisdom

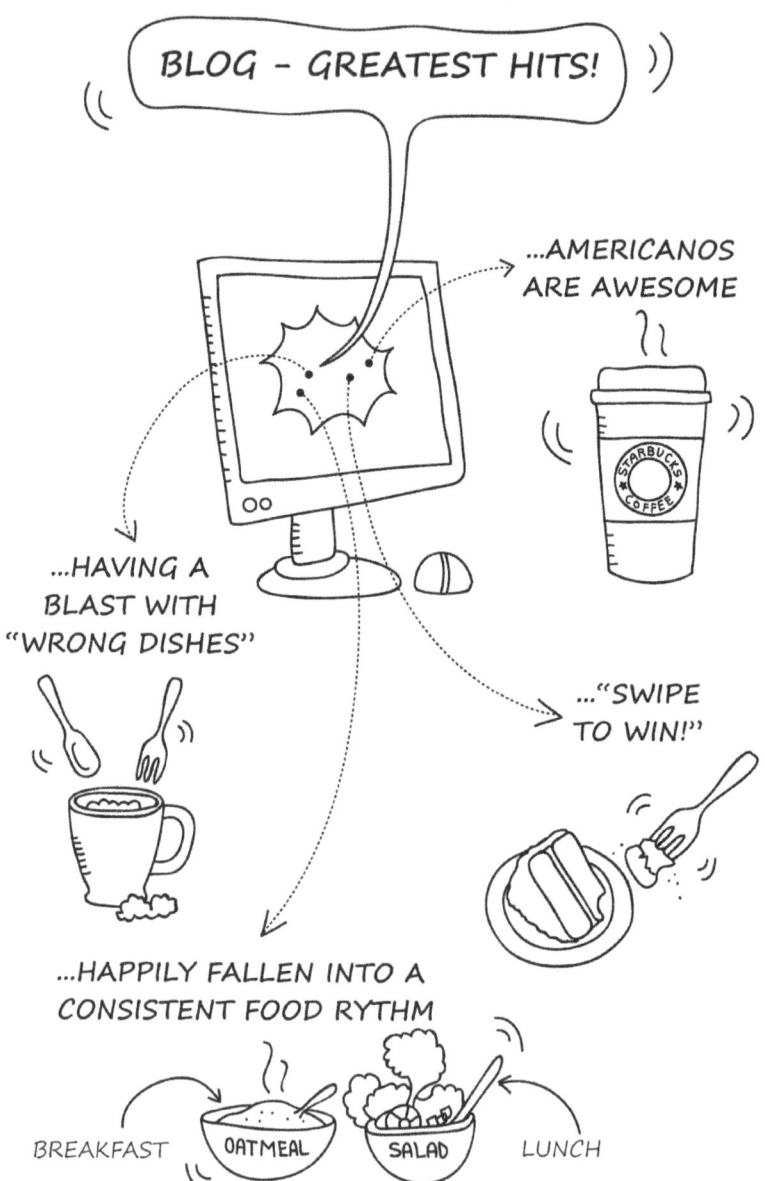

Simple Guy BLOG Wisdom

As time marches on, so do the posts on the Simple Guy website. I thought it would be good to share some of the thoughts and emotions I had while in my first six months of weight loss, as well as my thinking and observations in the years that followed...

GENERAL BLOG POSTS:

+ I am still surprised on the rare occasion when I look in the mirror... not only by my loss of weight, but also that I have been successful in doing so

+ My Starbucks americanos are still very important to me... so much so, that when I am in a restaurant or at home, I am having hot tea which makes my Starbucks run even more special

+ I am having a blast using the "wrong dishes" when I eat. Many times I will use coffee mug at home rather than a bowl... or in a self service place or a place where we are served "family style", I am using a saucer or a coffee cup to replace a full size plate or a bowl

+ Missing meals or not eating my usual things seem to get me slightly off track. I find the greatest success to starting my day off with a very small bowl of oatmeal and then just stick to MY plan has been the best strategy (for me)

+ My love for cold cereal (and was my "go to option" for a fast dinner) is totally gone. With the exception of a shot of Grape Nuts in my morning oatmeal... or in some yogurt at night

+ BREAD COUNTS! Somehow, as Americans, we have wrongly come to believe that bread doesn't count when we think about our food intake. We will talk about the turkey sandwich and what a good choice it was... but what about the bread? Also, let's not forget that bread usually brings along some of it friends... like butter for toast, mayo on a turkey sandwich, or a heap of PB&J. Bread may look like a nice guy, but many times he is like a bad relative that you just can't get rid of... so start being creative, reduce your bread intake and let the weight loss begin!

+ Now that I am down around 20 pounds, I also think that my posture is better. I am not sure that it actually is, but I seem more conscious of being more "upright"

+ Finish strong!! One thing that I have learned is when I do eat out, make my last bite a great one. I reserve some of the best things from my order to have my last bite be my best

+ Own it!! Once you lose your first 5 pounds... you need to feel like you "own" that weight and are not going back. You should be at that weight or lower for a week to have full ownership; then focus to lose the next five... once there, own that number. Hitting a "target weight" is good... but without "owning it", it will just be a moment in time

+ Before the SG, going to bed was the most anticipated part of my day; but now, bedding down is a bit of a downer as I can not wait to get rollin' the next morning

+ According to my wife and kids, I rarely snore... which certainly WAS NOT the case before my weight loss

+ I have the opportunity to work with some awesome people. One gal, about my age has boundless energy and focus. Not sure how she does it, but I bet part of it is that she eats right, as my energy and my ability to "fire up" in the morning has been a noticeable and dramatic change

+ Here is a Japanese concept which can certainly pertain to our food consuming life as well. KAIZEN: Small improvements made every day will lead to a massive improvement overall. Love it!

+ This is kooky... now I have happily fallen into a rhythm of food consistency/regularity (oatmeal for breakfast and a medium salad bar serving for lunch). I find myself only wanting the same things for each meal. Before I met the SG, I was fueled and energized by variety (Baskin Robbins, Noah's bagels, TGI Fridays...), but now places like this feel somewhere between distracting and overwhelming. I am really liking my simplistic, repetitive pattern... as it too, has made my life less fussy

+ For some reason I have started to try and do a bit of "ab work". I have this goofy roller-thing that my wife bought on an infomercial (OK, maybe I bought it, but it was years ago)... so now I do just 12 in the morning and 12 in the evening (the first time I did 25 I was crazy-sore for 3 days!). Not sure if it will do anything...but at least it will satisfy my urge to "try"...

+ My "enough" is now noticeably less than when I started the SG lifestyle. Smaller portions are what I crave... big portions of anything seem to live somewhere between "wrong and just plain bad"

+ As my portions have become smaller, I find myself gravitating to smaller pates and bowls to put my food on. My full-sized bowls and plates in my kitchen are now rarely used (by me)

+ The next time you are at a fast food place, pretend like Obie Wan is looking at you as if you were a storm trooper, gently waving his hand and saying, "This is not the food you are looking for... move on"

+ Somehow my new beverage of choice is a cup of water with no ice and just a splash of 7-Up. It may sound weird, but for me, it is way better than just water... and way better for me than a soft drink

+ I have never been a big salad guy till I started rollin' with the Simple Guy. Before quantity was a requirement of each meal... but now, being super selective at a salad bar and making a small (or at least smaller) masterpiece is really working well for me

+ I seem to have lost interest in fast food burgers... rarely going there anymore... except with my teenage son. I wonder (when I was hooked on McDonald's for the first 3- 4 months) if this was just a natural need to stay connected to my eating past... the food... the ordering process... the tray... the surroundings... it is certainly a mystery to me

+ My weight has stabilized... even with more regular indulgences

+ Portioned and infrequent indulgences: 1 (not 2 or 3 like before) donuts every couple of weeks... a small piece of bread to dip into olive oil at an Italian restaurant

+ Fork fulls to win! I have found that a fork is a pretty darn handy way to indulge. It serves as an excellent "portion control devise". If I decide to have a little piece of brownie... before grabbing a square, I now use a fork and my only decision is if I'm going to have one or two fork fulls... eat it, love it and walk away

+ Most of us have heard the term, "cheat to win"... but for the Simple Guy, I have now adopted the philosophy of "Swipe to Win." By successfully swiping (with permission, of course) a couple of bites of my wife's sweet potatoes or a fork full of her dessert... this gives me a wonderfully satisfying taste of my eating past without being confronted with entire portion to (likely mis-) manage myself

+ OK, full disclosure. After a couple of weeks I gave up on the ab-roller thing. I still hate myself for buying it, but I am too cheap to get rid of it... my bad.

+ A better fast food option for me (at this moment) is Taco Bell (for me, it's not about the food there... it's their darn hot sauce that I crave). One "fresco taco" with hot sauce is so sinfully good. Never be fooled... tortillas are evil... even the little ones!! Make this a weekly treat at most

+ Still nothing seems worth having in the Starbucks treat case... although I still go to Starbucks about 10 times a week for my tall americano. There have been times when I purchased a single banana... I always wondered who bought bananas there...

+ I was rollin' for a while by having the barista add foam to my americano (a tall foamy americano if you want to try one). That was great for a couple of months, but I have now bounced back to one without foam

+ My daily ritual of high cocoa content chocolate has mysteriously ended. I am not sure what the insight is here, but it is clear that some cravings have "just ended"

+ Ready for my next run to Goodwill. I have a pile of clothes (now shirts are included) that were "on the bubble" with regard to fit and size... now, I have no interest in keeping them

+ Still no running for the Simple Guy, but my tennis racquet is re-strung and I have had several (very fun) "social hits" a couple times a month

+ Oatmeal = control!! I now find myself taking my (stupid) instant oatmeal packets, a plastic spoon and crushed walnuts when I travel for personal reasons. I do love oatmeal... but I also feel it gives me both control and a sense of protection from being victimized by whatever there might (and might not) be available for breakfast

+ I am really into drinking warm water in the morning and hot water with many of my meals

+ Holy smokes... I just went through the TSA line in the airport. When the agent handed me back my license, I noticed that my weight was lower than stated... for the first time in 20 years I won't need to "round down" my weight when I renew my license!

+ People seem to always ask me if I have more energy since I lost the weight. In general, I would say no... although maybe I do, but since the change was so darn gradual, I just have not been able to tell

+ This is weird, but I seem to wake up an hour earlier (new for me) AND at full speed (REALLY NEW for me). This is indeed a change... and I must say, one of the best outcomes of my weight loss!!

+ I am still living in the halo of accolades about my visible weight loss. I wish I had something more magical to tell them... but really, for me, it is nothing more than hangin' with the Simple Guy

+ Here is a bad thing to say... but I am finding it more and more true, "Food is pissing me off!!" I seem to get grumpy when many meetings and most invitations to be with friends and family seem to have food as the centerpiece. I almost wish someone would declare a day of the week or a week a month when food could not be part of any gathering. I enjoy socializing and I also attend a lot of meetings... I love them both, but I feel like my will power is constantly being tested, and that gets me grumpy

+ Beer has fallen off my radar... really not sure why... but my interest is near zero

+ After about six months, things that were indulgences before (a big milk shake, a vanilla bean frappiccino, a peanut buster parfait at Dairy Queen) seem to be nearly impossible consumption items now. I am not trying not to want them... they just don't hold the same "temptation value" as in the past

+ I am becoming a bit of a "label-looker". In the past, I rarely looked at the nutrition facts; as frankly, I was just not interested. I still am not. However, now I do give it the occasional glance to how it rates with carbohydrates. When you're not sure about what you might be ready to consume, a quick look is a pretty darn good thing to do. I ended up with a little... and I mean little box of raisins and thought, "This MUST be a healthy choice... they're raisins". Once I checked the facts, I realized that little box had

10% of my daily carb value! I took a pass, but in the past would have happily consumed the box in a bite or two

+ Imagine a world where: eating free samples at the store cost you money... you had to pay a fee for owning clothes that no longer fit you... but, every time you choose to walk rather than drive, you get paid. Taking the thinking a step further, imagine: every soda you drink cost you $10.... every individual fast food item you order cost you $10 (so a burger, fries and a drink would cost you $30). I love the dollar menu, but I wonder what I would do if each of the items on the menu we ten bucks a piece... When I think about it like that, I wonder if I crave the food or do I crave the value?

+ When dining out, do yourself a favor and have your menu item selected before you sit down. It is just too darn easy to have the chicken Caesar salad (you thought you were going to order) turn into mozzarella sticks and a personal pan pizza after staring at the menu!!

+ The big picture!! If you are anything like me, just starting to adjust my lifestyle around food was a real transition. My low-carb strategy continues to work great for me and I achieved my goal to lose about 20 unwanted pounds. If for some reason, this is just too big of a change, then set a lower goal of losing 5 pounds and keep it off for the calendar year... then the following year, do the same until you reach your target weight. For me, a couple of simple changes did the trick... but for you and your lifestyle, a super slow stair-step weight loss method may be the worth a try as the optimum way for you to control your weight. Remember, our weight is just a number... the real goal is our health, not the time it takes us to get there

+ When you go out and order a salad, remember these 5 words of wisdom, "Dressing on the side, please!"... it will be a game changer and keep YOU in total control

+ I used to not be satisfied till I was full... and I mean physically full... no room left. Now, on the rare occasion that I am stuffed, if feels both bad and just "wrong"

+ My dinner salads seem to be getting smaller and smaller over time. When I first started the Simple Guy Diet, my bowl was heaped with salad, and now, I bet my dinner volume is half of when I started. After the first year, I stopped adding meat to my salad for the most part. Adding flavors to my salad dressing (like a tablespoon of BBQ sauce) seemed to be like a new magic thing to do.

SIMPLE GUY STORIES:

+ I am a bit bummed out by the food consumption of others. I am certainly not a judgmental person, but I kind of feel that way when watching others eat. In a recent flight for work to Europe I sat next to 3 sisters (ages 60-70) flying over the Atlantic on vacation. My usual gig is to eat something I choose to eat at the airport and pass on the first meal on the plane. Within an hour of takeoff, a monster egg-salad sandwich and a big bag of Kettle Chips emerged from one of their carry-ons. They were like three wild dogs sharing their prey as they passed this monstrous mess back and forth to each other. Within the 90 minutes, our airplane meal came... I passed... and they consumed!! A round of raviolis, a dinner roll, cheese and crackers, a small salad with dressing and a brownie were licked clean. Gold stars for them!! Hours later I woke up from my nap and the food-sisters we knocking down a giant piece of chocolate cake they had carried on as well... this chocolate beast was about the same volume as a half a carton of cigarettes. Not a crumb survived. Our pre-landing omelet was met with the same enthusiasm... where does all the food go?... and man, am I THRILLED that I am not like that anymore!

+ Your weight is like flying a jet. I took a week off of work to have a little bonus family time. While off that week, it seems I had totally lost control of what food I was confronted with... and ultimately consuming! The days seemed to be focused around "favorite places to eat"... not to mention hanging with friends and family which too, made "eating right" tough for me. After the first several days of "bad behavior", my weight had not really changed... foolishly, I believed that my new life style had perhaps created the antidote for the consumption of guacamole and chips, pizza and peanut M & Ms. Near the end of my week-o-fun, my weight was hopping up about a pound a day. The following workweek I reverted back to my Simple Guy way of living. Equally foolish, I thought a day or two would do the trick... in reality it took another 5-8 days to get back and "own" my desired weight. The moral to the story is... you can't blow OR fix your weight in a single day... or two. The best analogy I can think of is that our weight is like flying a jet plane. It takes a while to get the plane rolling with enough speed to achieve liftoff... conversely, it takes a long time to slow a jet plane down. Any change, good or bad, will require you to have a longer (than you might think) runway of time to see results.

VACATION POSTS:

+ On our annual week-long vacation/family reunion, the chips, cookies and assorted kid-friendly boxed-snacks never got consumed... at least by me. Although a couple of red vines did find their way into my possession

+ I am still craving my daily oatmeal and grape nuts every morning. In fact I brought the stuff with me on the family get away... it was both comforting and helped me steer clear from the daily homemade scones and sticky buns

+ On vacation I had a blast playing golf several times... but also walking 6-10 miles (by choice) everyday... in fact, I couldn't get enough (OK, the weather was awesome)!! I am now an official "walkaholic"... not one of those goofy super fast guys or the dude carrying weights, but rather just walking "with a purpose"... about 18 minute miles... or 3.5 miles per hour

+ When traveling near or far, consider an omelet... pass on the toast and the potatoes... as a good "travel anytime meal" alternative

Be sure to check in from time to time on the Simple Guy BLOG... Simply by logging on to our website at:

www.simpleguydiet.com

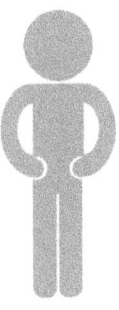

A Simple Summary

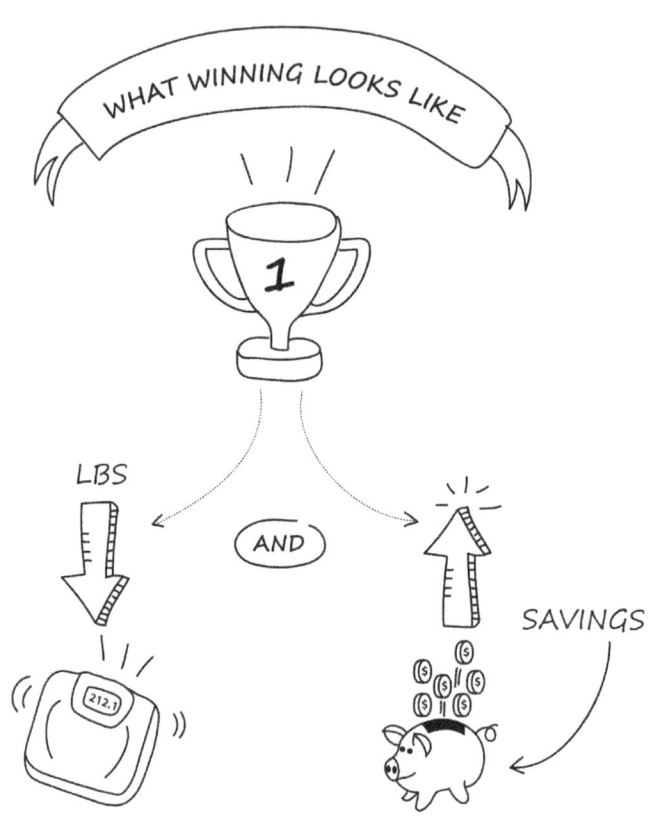

A Simple Summary

☐ Commit to 30 Days (dedicate a fixed amount of time)

☐ Buy a Digital Scale (your new "honest" friend)

☐ Have a Food Roadmap (a plan <u>you</u> can live with)

☐ Become a Genius Salad Maker (unique to you)

☐ Enjoy the View (get out the door and start movin'!)

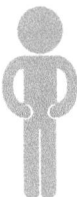

My brothers, <u>it is just this simple</u>!! Your toughest hurdle will be the "desire to lose weight" and the "will power to commit" (sadly) DO NOT come in the form of a pill that you can purchase... This is all on you!

The simpler you keep things, the easier the weight losing process will become. Just take control and dedicate yourself to 30 days and see what happens. I bet you will discover what I did and find that the Simple Guy Diet is indeed **A GREAT PLACE TO START!!**

About the Author

Skip Lei is a self-proclaimed pathetically average 50- something male with a job, a wife, two kids and a small yard to mow. Happily living in the Pacific Northwest, he gave up on weight loss and blamed an unfairly slow metabolism and a lack of commitment for his creeping weight. Realizing that most diet programs were too structured or too alien, he simply created his own life-style fitting method to see what would happen. He would be the first to admit that his weight loss story is not cosmic... he would also smile knowing he shed nearly 10% of his body weight and is no longer referred to as a "chubby-hubby".

About the Illustrator

Nitya Wakhlu is a graphic facilitator who has worked with Fortune 500 companies and social change-makers around the world. Nitya works with clients to transform complex ideas and strategies into simple visual tools that create clarity, engage people and drive action.

More of her work can be seen at www.nityawakhlu.com

Simple Guy Philosophy
BONUS SECTION

Now that we have tackled weight loss... here is all you need to do prioritize if you want to be REALLY happy in life. There can only be one #1, there can be no ties.

- *Where you live*
- *Your partner*
- *Your occupation*

As an example... if you had the right mate, you really wouldn't care as much about the other two, OR if you lived exactly where YOU wanted to live, would that be enough to bring you supreme happiness, OR if you were so passionate about your work/employer/compensation, would the other two would hold less value?

GIVE IT A THINK...

Please don't play this game if you are loaded with cash as you have likely used your financial ability to attempt to "buy it all". Feel free to use this as a table topic game at your next (hopefully) non-food gathering!! Simplifying your life in everything you do (including weight loss) is indeed the key to the kingdom!

NOTES

The reason we needed to have these final

NOTES

NOTES

publishing. I had the option to add

NOTES

additional content but refused; as the whole

NOTES

purpose of this book was to be simple and

NOTES

NOTES

write/capture meaningful notes, or just rip

NOTES

them out, cut them into little pieces and use

NOTES

as scrap paper to create grocery lists for

NOTES

the next four weeks…. Enjoy!

www.ingramcontent.com/pod-product-compliance
Ingram Content Group UK Ltd.
Pitfield, Milton Keynes, MK11 3LW, UK
UKHW022212230426
12048UKWH00016BA/803